Beyond Graves' Disease

Beyond Graves' Disease
Thoughts and Reflections

Celia Marie

Beyond Graves' Disease Thoughts and Reflections

This book is designed to provide accurate and authoritative information with regard to the subject matter covered. This information is given with the understanding that the author is not engaged in rendering legal, professional advice. Since the details of your situation are fact dependent, you should additionally seek the services of a competent professional.

Published in the United States of America

ISBN: 978-0-557-40914-3

1. Health & Fitness/Diseases/Immune System

2. Health & Fitness/Diseases/General

Dedication

I dedicate this book to all who have been diagnosed with Graves' disease. I challenge each of you to become an over comer of Graves' disease, moving Beyond Graves' and on to the endless possibilities that await you now that you have been forever changed. Share your stories and raise Graves' disease awareness. I salute you.

Acknowledgements

Maria, you have my deepest gratitude. I could have never made it without you. You have been there every step of the way, at every doctor's visit (there've been hundreds), every medical procedure, at the hospital during my surgery and at home. Your constant reminder of "I love you" on a daily basis pushed me when I was fed up with the battle. Your continual forgiveness each time I have blown it with you has been the fragrance that has made the most difficult times bearable. Ri, you have an amazing amount of compassion, cheerfulness and patience. I pray that you will always remember the time you told me "Mom, what this world needs the most is Jesus." Ri, you are God's mouthpiece in your generation. I am thankful that you were given to me as a gift from God. Continue to share your light and infectious laughter with the world!

I am thankful to Pat for providing the much needed medical insurance, paying for the co-pays and prescriptions. Thank you.

Thank you, Glynis. Your daily prayers, encouragement, phone calls, cards with a little something extra, all of the laughter, in addition to you listening to my heart more than my words has all been part of this journey. By the time this book releases we will have been friends for 25 years! I am amazed at how God could bring two women together who are so different and yet knitted together so closely; of course this goes much deeper than our mutual appreciation of "It's a Mad, Mad, Mad, Mad World" and "Anne of Green Gables." I love you, Glynis.

Introduction

August 2008

As I sat in the auditorium at Vineyard Church North Phoenix in August of 2008, I looked around at the congregation. My mind was wandering (which is not uncommon when you have Graves' disease) and then I looked back at Pastor Brian T. Anderson as I focused in on the words coming from his lips. "Your life is a book," he said, "you are the one who must decide if your book is going to be a good one or a great one."

For weeks my friend, Glynis, and I had been talking about the book I was planning to write. It all started out as a joke. One day I was pouring my heart out to her on the phone and I jokingly said that I should write a book about all of this and she bantered back that it would be on the bestseller list. Even though we talked about my book several times since that first conversation I began to ponder if that is what I was supposed to do. What if I was supposed to write about my journey with Graves' disease?

I had been involved in journalism since my junior high days. In senior high school I was a member of the Quill and Scroll Society, co-editor of our school newspaper, feature editor of same newspaper and after I graduated from college I began my 501C-3 called Pure Stoke Press. I wrote and published articles for extreme sports enthusiasts on topics of surfing, running, hiking, and skiing. My article "Climb the Mountain" was distributed at the annual walk for cancer at South Mountain in Phoenix, Arizona. My "Pure Stoke" article (for surfers) was given to surfers in Imperial Beach, Tourmaline Surfing Park and even found its' way to Hawaii. I also wrote an article on the Iditarod that was handed out at the Kuskokwim 300 dog sled race in Bethel, Alaska.

As my mind once again focused on the words that Pastor Anderson was speaking he said "In closing, it's up to you to decide if your life is going to be a good book or a great book." I began to think that I was not only supposed to write just one book, but a trilogy of my journey with Graves' disease. As the service was ending I prayed that if this was the path that God wanted me to take that He would let me know and give me the words to write.

May 2010

The book that you are about to read is the third book in my Graves' disease series. Part of me is hesitating to begin writing the first chapter because I know that this will be my last book in this series while another part of me is thrilled to begin writing this book. Many of you have read my books, *Life in the Cave Overcoming Grave's Disease* and *Emerging From the Cave Surviving Graves ' Disease.* Both of them focus on not only how Graves' disease has affected me but how it has also affected my family and friends.

My purpose in writing *Beyond Graves' Disease* is to share idioms, quotes and verses that have become meaningful to me upon discovering that I have Graves' disease which is treatable but not curable. My life has been forever changed. I have chosen to not give up but to go on. This choice was not easy. From the years 2005-2008 I bitterly fought all of the symptoms, went through the denial, the paralysis of fear, the deep pain, sorrow, and anger; yet, before my surgery there was a turning point where I made a conscious decision to choose to live and to not let the fear of living with Graves' disease rob me of a beautiful life filled with each new day of the wonder of the possibilities that lie ahead. I chose to live for my daughter's sake but what I've received is far much more than any expectations I had dreamed of and hoped for.

The words that you are about to read are vignettes of possibility, hope, light, dreams, laughter and surrender. I offer you the words of someone who doesn't dream that it's over. Limitless possibilities are my focus now.

1.

Never give in. Never give in. Never, never, never, never -- in nothing, great or small, large or petty--never give in, except to convictions of honor and good sense.

Winston Churchill

Many times I was tempted to give up during my battle with Graves' disease. Each time I was tempted to throw in the towel I would remember these wise words of Winston Churchill.

2.

Rome wasn't built in a day.

French Proverb

I really love this proverb because it reminds me to be gentle with myself. The important things in life take time. Your healing recovery may come in a split second but mine has been in the making for four years.

3.

"The LORD your God in your midst, The Mighty One, will save; He will rejoice over you with gladness, He will quiet you with His love, He will rejoice over you with singing."

Zephaniah 3:17

This verse became very special to me in September of 2009. During one of my daily devotions the Lord impressed upon me through my cognitive processes that although I was experiencing deep sorrow He was going to give me a new song (Psalm 40:3). I immediately thought of the above verse taking great comfort and immense joy in the promise that He is saving me, rejoicing in me as His precious daughter, calming me with His pure and perfect love along with rejoicing in me, His creation, with singing! This is very beautiful and precious to me that the Creator of the universe takes notice and delights in me. I am complete in this all-encompassing affirmation of my Heavenly Father.

4.

Be God's
Rich Mullins

This one is a challenge and my heart's deepest desire. I want to **"Be God's"** yet in order to truly do this I must choose to die to myself many times in the course of a day. If I am to be His I need to let go of my wants, wishes, and desires to be the vessel that He can use and flow through.

It is a very frightening thing to let go to **"Be God's"**. If you choose to do this please e-mail me at CeliaMarieAuthor@gmail.com and share your experience of how you've accepted Rich Mullins challenge to **"Be God's"**. I also welcome hearing from you if you are a fan of Rich Mullins. His songs are truly the soundtrack of my life.

5.

An apple a day keeps the doctor away.

Ancient Roman Proverb

The naturopathic approach to healing includes healthy eating. Apples are a source of Vitamin C which is good for our immune system. They also contain fiber and bioflavonoids.

6.

A merry heart does good, like medicine, But a broken spirit dries the bones.

Proverbs 17:22

Laughter is conducive to healing. Surround yourself around positive people. Go watch a comedy. Read a humorous book. Laugh at yourself. Listen to upbeat music with a positive message. Laugh at yourself. Yes, I repeated that on purpose!

7.

For I know the thoughts that I think toward you, says the LORD, thoughts of peace and not of evil, to give you a future and a hope.

Jeremiah 29:11

This is truly my life verse. I chose this while I was in college. I trust this promise completely. Do you have a life verse? Please e-mail me at CeliaMarieAuthor@gmail.com and share your life verse with me.

8.

Birds of a feather flock together.

16th Century Proverb

This is so true. Do you want peace in your life? Do you want Truth in your life? Do you want laughter in your life? Do you want stimulating conversation in your life? Seek peaceful, truthful, humorous, interesting people to spend your time with.

9.

And you shall know the truth, and the truth shall make you free.

John 8:32

It takes courage to seek the truth. When I was 33 I was on a serious quest for truth. I meant business and this quest took me to sitting in a chair across from Ellen, my counselor. She saw me weekly in the beginning because I was so distraught. She explained to me that my cup had overflowed and that was why I found a need to meet with her. She went on to say that she wished that victims like me would not be bound in the shame of what they had survived. She told me the truth. The truth was what happened to me was not my fault. She showed me that my abusers were affected by what they had done to me just as much as I was affected. Week after week, month after month we peeled back the layers of shame, humility, grief, and deep pain; gradually while we were stripping away every deception I was becoming a young woman experiencing true freedom for the very first time. Thank you, Ellen, and thank you God. I feel compelled to share that this verse literally means that Jesus Christ is the Truth and He truly makes us free. Through Jesus we have redemption and resurrection because He was wounded for our transgressions and by His stripes we are healed of any physical, spiritual, emotional or mental affliction we are either battling or have been freed of. He is God's gift of love to the world and whoever believes and accepts His son, Jesus Christ, as their personal Savior will have everlasting life.

10.

Forgiveness is the fragrance that the violet sheds on the heel that has crushed it.

Mark Twain

There is power, strength and beauty in forgiveness. Do you need to forgive someone today? Let the powerful healing of forgiveness set you free.

11.

Nothing great was ever achieved without enthusiasm.

Ralph Waldo Emerson

Think about your greatest achievements. Were you enthusiastic in your pursuit of your achievements? Your enthusiasm will realize great accomplishments.

12.

Follow your bliss.

Joseph Campbell

This is amazing. I have discovered that my God-given talents and abilities have led me straight to my bliss. I am thankful to God for the unique talents and abilities that He's given to me.

13.

Yet in all these things we are more than conquerors through Him who loved us. For I am persuaded that neither death nor life, nor angels nor principalities nor powers, nor things present nor things to come, nor height nor depth, nor any other created thing, shall be able to separate us from the love of God which is in Christ Jesus our Lord.

Romans 8:37-39

This promise has sustained me through the most difficult times of my life. I believe in this passage and know that this Truth has helped in my journey of healing with Graves' disease. I am not fully healed and there is no cure for Graves' disease but I have come so far in comparison to where I was when first diagnosed with Graves' disease in September of 2006.

14.

*The Lord bless you and keep you; the Lord
make His face shine upon you, and be
gracious to you; the Lord lift up His
countenance upon you,
And give you peace.*

Numbers 6:24-26

This blessing is my favorite. I look forward to
Pastor Brian T. Anderson speaking this over our
congregation. I soak in the peace, comfort and joy
that these words bring to give me nourishment for
the coming week.

Epilogue

June 2010

The 12 idioms, quotes and verses that I have shared with you all have special meaning to me. Of course I have many more but these stand out to me the most at this time in my life.

I thank you for joining me as I have shared my journey with Graves' disease in my books, *Life in the Cave Overcoming Grave's Disease, Emerging From the Cave Surviving Graves' Disease* and this book you're now holding in your hands *Beyond Graves' Disease Thoughts and Reflections.* I chose to not put my whole focus on the negative aspect of Graves' disease in this book because my perspective on my life at this point in the journey is recovery. I believe that we each have four components in our being: physical, spiritual, emotional and mental. I wanted to touch on each aspect within these pages. In order to be in balance we need to nuture each of these areas.

Further, I have surrendered my old life in exchange for my new life. I look forward to watching Maria, my daughter, carve out her own life with all our future moments of laughter, joy, hugs, failures, heart-to-heart talks, prayers, disagreements, misunderstandings and forgiveness that are on the horizon. I am excited about the plans that the Lord has for me and Maria.

My newest hobby is learning new languages. I also continue to enjoy social media sites including Facebook and Myspace.

I have discovered that my bliss is now the field of screenwriting. I am looking forward to this new chapter in my life as a screenwriter. I believe that we need quality films that focus on integrity, justice, education and faith. I would love to offer a quality film educating the public about Graves' disease.

I wish you the best in your journey with Graves' disease or any other disease from which you are recovering. Please e-mail me at CeliaMarieAuthor@gmail.com and share your story of recovery with me. I would love to hear from you.